Herbal Antibiotics

Top 15 Natural Herbal Home-Made Remedies to Cure Your Disease and Boost Your Immune System (Herbal Medicine, Holistic Healing, Autoimmune Solution)

By Carrie Dresden

Table of Contents

Disclaimer

This book should not replace the advice of your medical practitioner. It is very important to stay on track with medication your doctor has given you and to make sure that it does not conflict with current medication. If you are pregnant, please consult your doctor before following any advice, as every pregnancy is different. We do not accept any liability and we advise readers to consult a medical practitioner before following the advice in this book. Caution should always be taken in regards to health.

Introduction

If you find yourself constantly getting sick or battling illnesses, then you might need a little bit of an immune system boost! This can be easier to achieve than it sounds and there are plenty of things you can do at home to help you fight off diseases and improve your immune system. This is an important part of staying healthy and strong and should not be taken lightly.

In this book, we will talk about 15 ways to stay healthy and strong, ranging from practical tips to herbal remedies for all of your immune system needs. It is important to note that everyone is different and some remedies will work better for some people than others. However, most of these are proven to boost immunity, and it is a great way to ensure that you truly do get the most out of your health and your life while increasing your immune system.

So if you're sick of being sick, and the thought of medication does not appeal to you, then this might just be the book that you have been looking for! Packed full of important tips, easy to read tricks and good advice, you will have your health back to standard in no time!

Chapter 1: Practice Good Hygiene

At first, this probably does not seem like it is an herbal way of keeping healthy and technically, it is not. However, it is an organic, homemade way to protect your immune system and get strong. If you are suffering from diseases then this is a good way to prevent the spread and prevent yourself from getting secondary infections of diseases which can weaken your immune system, further and lead to a longer time fighting to get better.

It is a simple step that cannot be said often enough. Washing your hands is a vital way to ensure that you take care of yourself and keep yourself healthy. You should wash your hands several times a day, especially before eating or preparing food. This helps prevent the spread of infection and minimizes the chances that you will ingest unsightly diseases and germs. This is a great way to protect yourself and it is simple, cheap and free, which makes it a great option regardless of your budget, your time frame, or anything else.

Another time you should wash your hands is after sneezing or coughing. This is a good way to prevent the spread of germs. If you have been to public places, it does not hurt to wash your hands. In fact, this is a great precautionary measure to prevent yourself from growing sicker, strengthen your own immune system and minimize the chances of becoming ill on a more day to day level. This is a powerful trick, once that should be used often. If you have any doubts, just think about a number of places you touch, and how many people touch them. You are transferring their germs to yourself and this is not a great way to protect yourself and keep yourself safe like you need to. By taking this to heart, you increase the chances of keeping yourself healthy and free from germs and diseases on a day to day level.

Chapter 2: Use Garlic

Garlic is an amazing way to boost your immune system! Garlic is a natural way to enhance your own strength, immune system, and health, and it's not a very difficult way to do it! In fact, most people would argue that garlic tastes pretty great, which makes it a wonderful option and it is very hard to argue with it. There are many ways that you can consume garlic, and you will find that these remedies are fantastic for so many things. For example, you can simply take garlic on your food. By eating large amounts of garlic in your day to day life, you will reap the benefits of its amazing properties. If you do not typically enjoy garlic based foods, then simply eating a section of a clove of garlic can do wonders. Once clove of garlic per day is an amazing way of making sure that you truly do get the nutrients and immune boosting properties that you want and need.

If you cannot stomach garlic, or you work in an industry where the thought of having garlic breath would be terrible for your career, then you need to consider alternatives to this option. An alternative that works very effectively is taking garlic capsules. This gives you all of the benefits of garlic without any of the bad breath of sickness that you might feel if you do not like the taste of garlic, or if you are concerned about having bad breath constantly. Taking a supplement like this is a great way to make sure you have long-term good health. Be mindful of which supplements you choose, and make sure it is pure without any added problems. This is a good way to keep on top of your immune system.

So why is garlic so powerful? Garlic contains several great properties that help boost your immune system. It contains antiseptic properties and it helps to fight off infections. Essentially, garlic is a simple, effective and powerful way to boost your immune system and take control of your health.

Chapter 3: Black Currants Are Good!

If you are looking for something that you can easily slip into your everyday diet, then black currents are a great way to go. Black currents are very tasty, which makes them easy to eat. They are sweet and can be added to a number of different food items. They can be eaten with cereal, they can be eaten in a smoothie or you can eat them in pies. You can also eat them alone, and some sweet curries. They are a great way to boost your immune system and to ensure that you get the nutrients that you need in order to function well and effectively through your life.

Black currents are not too hard to find, and there are plenty of ways that you can enjoy them, a few of which we mentioned above to give you a head start. However, there are plenty of others ways to ensure that you get the intake that you need, and this includes the usage of cooking with them, or simply eating them plain if you like them. Both of these options are great, and they are pretty easy to slip into your daily diet without too much trouble. If you master this, then you will find an increase in health.

So what makes black currants so potent anyway? Well, black currants are great for boosting your Vitamin C intake, which is a fantastic way to boost immunity and health. They are also high in nutrients and there is some evidence that they can also help with the health of your eyes, which is a great investment!

Essentially, black currants are great for boosting your immune system, improving your nutrients intake and helping with your health. If you stay healthy, you will have a reduced chance of infections and diseases and this gives you a great head start on the healing process if you do ever get sick! If you are facing an illness, then an immunity boost is never a bad thing, after all!

Chapter 4: Flaxseeds and Healthy Nuts

A great item to keep in your cupboard is flaxseed! Flaxseeds are amazing at boosting your immune system and ensuring that your health is in great shape. Not only are flaxseeds known for improving your health, but they are rich in nutrients, which boost the immune system and give you the health increase that you need! Not only that but flaxseed taste great and they are amazingly easy to include in anything that you eat.

You can cook with flaxseed, or just eat them plain, whichever you prefer. The options are endless and you can do whatever you need to in order to ensure that you have the great time that you deserve in your life. These seeds are great for decreasing your chance of disease and in increasing your health and immune system strength. All in all, this is an amazing way to ensure that you keep on top of your health and diet. They are not too hard to include and can be added together with other items on this list, such as blackcurrant in order to ensure that you get the dietary needs you need in one easy to eat trail mix type package. No matter your preference for food, we know it is a simple way to make things work for you!

Flaxseed is very good at preventing a number of different diseases and infections and is fantastic for helping you to improve your health and the immune system no matter your age and stage, and this is a powerful and important way to make sure that you stay on top of your game at all times!

Chapter 5: Turmeric and Good Spices

If you are looking for a powerful spice that does it all, the turmeric is a great way to start! Since it is a spice it very easy to add to your cooking. You do not have to worry about struggling to eat it on its own. Simply add turmeric to your evening meals or your lunch and you are all set. It has a fantastic amount of good properties and is perfect for boosting your immune system and working to make you strong and disease resistant. It is a helpful preventative measure when it comes to diseases as well as infections and other nasty surprises. It is a great way to combat inflammation, and there are studies that claim it can help with arthritis, Alzheimer's and cancer.

It is a very powerful spice and it should be included in your daily diet whenever possible. There are turmeric supplements available if you struggle to take the spice, or if you find that it is too much for you. If you dislike the taste, then a supplement can be a great alternative and a fantastic way to make sure that you are taking the amount of spice that you need. It is a great way to boost your immune system and is a relatively easy and cheap way to do so, which is a perfect way to ensure that you achieve the results that you desire, and increase your health in the process.

It is also a pretty tasty spice, which makes it the perfect addition to so many meals and options that it is not even funny. This makes it a great addition to your daily intake!

Chapter 6: Water Intake

While this is technically not an herbal technique, it is a great way of keeping on top of your health and ensuring that you get the water intake that you need. Drinking water is an amazing way to ensure that you truly do get the immune system boost that you need and deserve.

Dehydration has a huge number of negative consequences and effects. It can lead to health issues and even death if you are not careful. Kidney damage is a common problem for dehydration suffers, and you need to be mindful of the effects that dehydration can have on you. It is important to keep up your water intake constantly. It is recommended that you have about eight glasses per day, but this is not a concrete figure. It is important to drink more if it is hot, or if you are engaging in physical activity above your usual level. If you keep yourself hydrated then you are sure to feel much, much better and have the increased strength and immunity that you deserve. This is a powerful way to engage in your own personal at home immune booster.

The great thing about drinking water is that you can do it no matter where you are! You can drink water at the shops, at a friend's house, on holiday, or at home! There is nothing you need to remember to bring in order to access water, and this is a great and effective way to ensure that you boost your immune system on a daily basis and protect yourself against diseases. The increase in health that you get from taking care of yourself and drinking more water cannot be stated enough. It decreases your chances of dehydration and improves your health, making this a very worthwhile cause to partake in!

Chapter 7: Eat Well

Eat a balanced diet. This is probably the most obvious of all of the options that we are listing, but it is vital to eat a healthy and balanced diet at all times. Eating a balanced diet does wonders for your immune system and is an amazing way to truly take in the glorious foods that we have around us.

So how can you eat healthily? Eating healthily starts off with eating more fruit and vegetables, which is a fantastic start to eating well. When you increase your intake of fruit and vegetables you increase your immunity and the ability to fight off any diseases and infections. This increased immunity is an amazing way to stay in tune with yourself and truly build your body up. Fruit and vegetables should be consumed frequently and with variety. It does not help your body to consume only one sort of healthy food constantly. The variety and balance are part of what makes a healthy diet so healthy. This is a powerful way to get a head start on your health and improve your immune system fairly easily.

If you are interested in making sure that your diet is truly balanced, then you need to look into other aspects, such as foods that you should not eat in excess. Sugary food is not good for a constant consumption, and you need to make sure that you do not eat too much of these types of food. It is also important that you do not eat foods that are excessively high in salt or other preservatives.

You must balance your choices with complex carbs and protein, however, you choose to ensure you get it. This balance is a great way to make sure that you really do eat the right food, and get the immunity boost that you love. This is important as immunity boosts that come from long term dietary changes are often the strongest.

This help fight against diseases and assist in boosting the immune system. If you make sure to take care of yourself in this way, you will most likely find that the positive effects on yourself and on your body are amazing and works as a highly effective trade off. Eating well consistently does wonders to prevent many diseases, help speed up recovery from current ones and improve on a range of different aspects of your life, making it a great choice!

So if you are looking for a very effective way to boost you immune system to a whole new level, this might just be the way to go!

Chapter 8: Green Tea

It is a very well-known fact that green tea is amazing for increasing your health. If you drink tea or coffee, consider substituting it for green tea. It is a great way to make sure you get the antioxidants that you need, and the health benefits are amazing. Even just one cup per day can do wonders for your health and for your immune system.

Drinking green tea dates back hundreds of years and there are no known negative side effects of drinking moderate amounts of the tea. It is a fantastic way to increase your intake of nutrients and antioxidants and boost your immune system. If you are looking for an easy, cheap and very effective way of boosting your immune system, then this is most certainly it! With high levels of nutrients and immune boosting properties, this is a great way to really get into your health.

The benefits of green tea are endless and luckily it is not hard to get a hold of it. A simple look at your local supermarket will prove to be highly effective in ensuring that you get the quality tea you need to boost your immune system fast! It doesn't have to be a big change, but lots of little changes can do wonders to ensure that you are healthy and can fight off potential diseases and infections that might be causing you pain or distress. Simple immune boosters like this are wonderful for making sure that you stay on top of your health in the best way!

Chapter 9: Yogurt

Probiotic foods are a great source if immune boosting properties. By making sure that you boost your immune system this way, you are protecting yourself from a host of different things that you do not get from most other types of immune boosters. This includes the prevention of stomach and intestine infections and the protection from respiratory infections. Probiotics are great because they boost the healthy bacteria found in your stomach and intestines. If you are on antibiotics due to problems or diseases, then this is a fantastic way to help regulate your stomach and help ease any trouble you have been having. It is also an amazing way to deal with a multitude of different issues, such as a low immunity.

So if you find that you're feeling a bit under the weather, or your immune system is taking a dive, increasing your intake of foods that contain probiotics is an amazing way to get on top of things. Of course, as with most things, it is important to ensure that you take these in moderation, so as not to overload your gut with too many bacteria. The balance here is the key, as it is with most immune boosting foods. Taking it in moderation is a wonderful way to feel better. Yogurt, for example, can be taken along with black currents, which makes for a fantastic snack that has huge immunity-boosting powers.

So if you are looking for a simple, yet very effective way to boost your own immune system and really take charge of what you are doing, then this might just be a good starting point. Remember, though, everything in moderation!

Chapter 10: Mushrooms

Mushrooms are a great way to make sure that you boost your immunity! They can be eaten alone, or put in with your cooking, and it is a great way to bring health into your diets. Japanese mushrooms are especially high in antioxidants and do wonders for the health and wellbeing of your body.

Antioxidants are amazing at really boosting the immune system, so foods that are rich in them are great. If you are sick or battling with diseases, then this is an amazing way to make sure that you stay up to date and on top of your health. A really great side note is the fact that they taste amazing. You can do a wonderful meal with these, and it is a great way to increase the flavor and truly get a taste of Japan into your cooking.

At the same time, the health benefits are endless, and it is a win-win situation in every way. The increased nutrients are a wonderful way to increase your immune system and help you lead a healthy life. Of course, the benefits go on a one, with increased immunity from diseases and infection, higher chances of being able to fight off current infections and diseases, and so, so much more. It is an important thing to think about and you should ensure that you take this into account.

Eating these foods will give you a big boost that will serve you well in regards to your health, mood, immune system and so, so much more!

Chapter 11: Zinc

Zinc is an amazing source of strength for the immune system. It is a great way to really increase your health in a simple and easy way. Eating foods that are rich in zinc is an amazing addition to your diet. Zinc can be found in many foods, such as crab and red meat. You need to ensure that you keep your zinc intake up and do not let it slip.

If you do not like foods that are rich in zinc, or cannot have them, then it is a good idea to take a zinc supplement in order to ensure that you stay healthy. The properties of zinc are fantastic and it is such a great way to really enjoy life and enjoy the health that you have.

If you are sick, zinc is a good way to help boost recovery and prevent you from getting secondary diseases, so it's a fantastic start to any healthy routine. So next time you are wondering where to start, this is a great place. It is easy, effective and if you can eat the foods we listed, it is very, very tasty too! With plenty of nutrients, these pack a punch and zinc is a simple, effective and very easy way to get on top of this without much fuss.

Zinc is necessary for development of immunity and to ensure that there is an effective growth in your body. This helps to fight diseases and so, so much more, making it a great way to watch your health, increase immunity and enjoy yourself while doing it!

Chapter 12: Vitamin D

Vitamin D boosts the immune system so, so well! This is a great way to really improve your ability to take in nutrients and is vital in development. So how can you organize yourself and get this done? Well, to be frank, a great way to do this is to simply get out there and go into the sunshine! The sunlight is an awesome source of vitamin D, and can help you in so many ways.

The great thing is that sunlight is free and that you can have all the sunlight you want! A little bit of sunlight every day gives you the vitamins that you need to improve your immune system and help promote growth. Sunlight is fantastic and very easy to come by.

Of course, you must be careful when it comes to sunlight. Being out too long in the sun can be damaging and have negative effects. Sunlight is great for you, but you need to be careful and be sure that you are exposed to it in moderation instead of in huge amounts. A great way to go about it is to make sure you put on sunblock constantly and that you go out into the sun for shorter periods of time, in order to make sure that you do not have any sort of problems with the sun, and that you do not damage your skin or body by taking part in this.

Moderation and precaution are great ways to ensure that you do not get sunburst, or damage yourself because of the sun. If you are very careful, you will find that you have the time you need to get the sun, vitamin D, and all the good effects. The effects of vitamin D include a big boost to the immune system and better absorbing of minerals and vitamins.

Chapter 13: Quit Vices

Now, this is not a herb at all, but it is just so important to keeping the immune system strong! This is a vital part of ensuring that you truly do get the health that you need. Smoking can cause a myriad of different illnesses and diseases, so if you smoke, it is very important to consider cutting down. If you do not smoke, take this as a warning and never start. It decreases the strength of your immune system and damages your health activity, leaving you sick and unable to cope will future illness.

Alcohol, while not quite as bad as smoking, should still be limited and heavily moderated. By limiting alcohol intake you will ensure that you boost you immune system instead of tearing it down and making yourself sicker. If you stick to this type of program, you will find that your health increases. If you are sick, you will find that this is a great way to keep yourself healthy and ensure that you heal. If you are not sick, this will help to prevent a ton of different issues. By simply cutting down on things such as smoking and drinking, you increase your chances of being healthy and you decrease your chances of being sick.

This is a great trade off, and you will feel much, much better too, regardless. This is important, as your personal health and wellbeing is the most important thing that you have. This is a great way to really step up your health and improve not only your immune system but your life!

Chapter 14: Exercise

This is not exactly a herb, but exercise is a very important part of having a strong immune system. If you are very sick, then it is important to do as many light and gentle stretches as you can. Do not push yourself, but be as active as your life allows at the moment. This is a great way to make sure that you have the active lifestyle that you need in order to stay healthy. Being healthy is such an important part of life, and should not be understated.

When you are healthy, your body is more apt to handle difficult things and it can make sure that you bounce back from illness far more quickly than before.

You do not have to push yourself to exhaustion, as this is not healthy either. It is simply important to make sure that you keep on track with your activity and that you do some movement every day, even if it is only something small. Activity has been shown to improve health and boost the immune system significantly. This is a great way to make sure that you have the high-quality immune system that you deserve, with high levels of health and a strong body. By doing this you will minimize the likelihood of infection, disease and sickness and boost recovery time and immune system. So if you are looking for a cheap and effective way to make sure that you boost your immune system and well and truly make a positive change for your health, then this is most certainly the way to go to achieve your goals and make them a reality!

Chapter 15: Get Good Sleep

Sleeping well is something that is often underestimated in regards to how very effective it is in terms of healing and immune system. If you do not get enough sleep, your immune system plummets. It can have devastating effects on your immune system and your overall health. The most important thing that you can do for your personal health is to ensure that you sleep properly and take good care of yourself in all ways.

Making sure that you get enough sleep is a wonderful way to make sure that you are on a good page and that your immune system is strong and healthy, just like the rest of you. If you are sick, sleeping is a good way to allow your body to heal itself and will give you the strength that you need to improve your body and overcome your illness. In fact, it is a very powerful tool when it comes to healing and it should be harnessed without hesitation. It is too easy to make sure that you get all of your work done and sacrifice sleep in the process but this is a bad idea and can damage your health and make it impossible to get anything done.

By taking care of yourself and ensuring that you get the sleep you need, you will be able to fight diseases and prevent your body from falling ill to a large extent. Sleeping is a wonderful way to boost your immune system. Take care not to sleep too long, but do not sleep too little. Getting the right about of sleep for your body, and your personal needs is a very powerful way to ensure that your health stays on track!

Conclusion

This book should not replace the advice of your medical practitioner. It is very important to stay on track with medication your doctor has given you and to make sure that it does not conflict with current medication. If you are pregnant, please consult your doctor before following any advice, as every pregnancy is different. We do not accept any liability and we advise readers to consult a medical practitioner before following the advice in this book. Caution should always be taken in regards to health.

It is important that you do what is best for your own personal health and always use safety. Your health and immunity are very important and you should always do what you can to care for it and boost it, whether you are feeling sick or not! Good luck in your health journey.